Table of Contents

Introduction from the Fat Loss Queen

Congratulations! I am so excited and feel privileged you chose to go with my fat loss program. You made a tremendous leap towards your health and wellness goals just by taking this first step.

You will learn to replace old ineffective habits with new healthy habits and choices that will pave the way to success for a new healthy lifestyle that will last a lifetime. This is NOT something you will do for a short time and then go back to old habits.

My 30-day program is going to offer you a **fast start** to a new lifestyle and help you achieve a level that can be maintained once the actions steps are taken and new habits are built. You will see results immediately. By the end of 30 days you will be the master of your own health, life and choices.

The Benefits of Burning FAT

Rapid fat loss is not safe for your health. It is a healthier way of life that will allow you to work towards burning fat hour-by-hour, day-by-day and week-by-week is much healthier. You will learn how to:
Make better choices
Look better
Feel better and confident in your self and your life
Have enough energy to carry you through the day
Remove the emotional barriers, pain and shame that keeps you from achieving your goals
Remain motivated at all times and put your health ahead every day of your life

The Fat Loss Queen Mind Set
Fat Loss Court Rules

"You become what you think about"
Earl Nightingale

You have to believe before your belief materializes in the physical plane.

- Fat Loss Queen

FAITH

Mind-set matters because all creation starts in our mind first before it can become a reality. This includes your life, choices and actions.

The vision of your new FLQ life style filled with ultimate health and vitality will create a burning desire and belief for your new life ahead. You will deliberately incorporate new choices and actions into your life.

As a Fat Loss Entourage Partner, these are the principles and tools you will abide by to get and maintain successful results:

1. **Take one day at a time and one week at a time.** This is how we will measure your advancement in your new Fat Loss life.

2. **Weigh yourself once a week on the same day and at the same time**. No more daily weigh-ins on the scale at home, grocery store or pharmacy. You must have a set day of the week that you weight yourself and take your waist measurement. It takes time to change habits that have been ingrained into your daily life.

3. **Avoid self-criticism** during this period of adjustment no matter what it takes - you have made the decision to change your life the FLQ way and you must stick with it. Way to go!

4. **Do NOT give up.**

5. **Do not compare yourself to others** in the program for friends who did the same program with different results. Everyone has a different metabolism and respond differently to specific foods and exercise but any action needs to have a plan to achieve the intended outcome.

~ FLQ PROGRAM MOTTO ~
WE WILL HELP YOU GET THE INTENDED RESULT

There really is a big difference between knowing what to do, doing what you know and being consistent. Knowledge is only half the battle. My patients tell me they know what to do, have read all the popular diet books and have been in all the popular weight loss programs.

My patients tell me that they know every thing they should. They have read all the popular diet books and have been in all the popular weight loss programs. But it is the "doing" part that most of you have trouble with and goals are what connect knowledge with action. Let's take a look at the "mind-set" part of the program.

FLQ TIPS TO A FAST START

1. **FLQ accountability log** – You must have a friend to help you succeed as accountability is the "X" factor for your FLQ program. Even though we call it a Fat Loss Program, it is basically a health for life system. Your intention is not to lose 15 pounds and be done with it and jump right back to your old habits.

The accountability log is a good way to track your day-to-day progress and the progress throughout the whole program. It keeps you accountable to the most important daily FLQ Fat to Fit steps. We will begin by recording your vitals including height, weight and body fat percentage that will serve as a baseline.

2. **Do NOT skip breakfast**. This is a must and non-negotiable. You may think you feel fine without breakfast or feel sick afterwards and simply eat a light lunch and big dinner. This will not help you lose body fat.

Did you know your brain thrives on glucose to get you through the day? After almost 8 hours of fasting during sleep, how do you expect your body to get up raring to go? How can you help your brain to focus and function throughout the day? If you have trouble with eating solid food for breakfast, you should have a protein shake instead.

Your brain uses glucose as fuel and to kick-start the day, it is absolutely necessary that you have breakfast. There has to be some carbohydrate with a good protein in your breakfast. (See the recipe section for ideas for morning smoothies).

3. **Make sure you take supplements daily** – your body's system is going through a major physiological change during fat loss and with the daily grind, responsibilities and lack of time, we tend to overlook out body's need for micronutrients. You have to adjust to the physiological changes occurring by addressing your body's needs. It is imperative to supplement your day with the supplements listed below:

A good-quality comprehensive Multi vitamin
Calcium and magnesium (500 mg. calcium/250 mg. magnesium)
Vitamin D3
Please note: Supplements are just that: they don't replace good nutrition.

4. **Drink Water** – this is one of the most important steps. Water is necessary for every process in the body. Drinking enough water is absolutely essential for burning fat and developing muscles.
60% of our body is made up of water
Our blood is 90%water
Bones have 20% water
Muscles are 70% water.
Hence, water is the most important nutrient on your journey to Fat Loss. The effects of dehydration are often very subtle.

TIP: The next time you get up in the morning and feel drowsy or tired during the day – drink some water because you are most likely dehydrated.

5.**Make movement a part of your life** – find an exercise you enjoy doing and look forward to. Make exercise a part of your daily regimen. You would not think of NOT brushing your teeth or taking a shower each day and you must think of exercise in the same way.

TIP: Lift weights – the more muscle you have, the more calories you burn just sitting here reading this book. It is an active tissue that requires energy and good quality protein to sustain itself.

Nutrition - The FLQ Way

One of the most commonly asked questions I receive from my clients are "What should I eat?" or "I eat only a little bit of food - Why am I gaining weight?" No doubt these are some of most defining parts of the program. Let us briefly review the most important nutrients.

Nutrients

Complete mini-meals every 3-4 hours is the key to successful weight loss and for maintaining that weight loss long term. It is important to make sure you are eating the right amount of protein, fats and carbohydrates so you will not feel deprived or store body fat. Choosing foods that heal rather than harm the body will give you a lifetime of health and automatic weight loss. You will be able to:
Control your appetite
Reduce stress and inflammation in the body
Turn calories into energy
Fortify your thyroid
Love your liver
Keep the following formula in mind every day when it is time to eat a mini-meal. This will open the door for you to achieve ultimate health and vitality and more importantly successful long-term weight loss. Simple, real, whole, nourishing foods will give your body what it needs to thrive and become fully alive.

50% CARBOHYDRATES of every meal should be carbohydrates like fruits, vegetables, whole grains, basically anything in the produce section or from the earth. Half your plate should be vegetables and you should limit your fruit servings to 2 per day. Good carbohydrates like those found in their natural state are needed for your brain to function and for consistent energy throughout the day. Bad carbohydrates are basically those found in the center aisles of the grocery store usually containing hydrogenated fats and high fructose corn syrup that are culprits to weight gain. Carbohydrates are made from plants and are called so because they have carbon and hydrogen in them. The main role of carbohydrates in our body is to maintain stabilized blood glucose levels in the blood.

25% PROTEIN of every meal should be good quality protein choices like chicken, turkey, fish, tuna, egg whites with one egg, buffalo, venison, good quality soy or whey protein. They are needed to support lean muscle tissue because the more muscle you have, the more calories you burn just sitting here reading this article. Plus you will stay full longer and it will slow down the digestion process of the carbohydrates.

25% FAT of your meal should include good fats like olive oil, nuts, seeds, avocados, macadamia nut oil, walnut oil or canola oil. Good fats are liquid at room temperature while most bad fats are solid at room temperature. Fat is needed by the body to transfer all the vitamins and minerals into the cells and tissues so you benefit from the nutrients ingested. Good fats like Omega 3's found in fish help reduce inflammation and are needed for healthy skin, hair, liver and kidney function.

YOUR GOAL (should you choose to accept it) is to consume 300-400 calorie whole-food meals every 3-4 hours.

This will:

    Increase your metabolism and turn you into a fat-burning machine instead of a fat-storing machine

    Keep you full all day by stabilizing blood sugar levels

    Make you feel satisfied, not deprived, hungry or starved!

    Give your body the nutrients it needs from WHOLE FOODS!

FLQ Menu Suggestions

FLQ plate
50/25/25 rule

Eating whole foods as opposed to highly processed foods will work with your body to ignite its natural fat-burning furnace, actually re-program it so your body will burn fat and keep it off for good. Eating the wrong foods will send messages of weight gain and disease to your body. By eating the right foods every day, you will send instructions of weight loss and good health to your body.

Breakfast suggestions:

Breakfast Burrito

Take 1 egg and 3 egg whites and scramble in a teaspoon of olive oil. Heat a brown rice tortilla in tin foil in the oven at 300 degrees for 5 minutes. Place the egg white mixture on top of the warm tortilla and top with 3 tablespoons of salsa.

(274 calories, 14 grams protein, 17 grams carbohydrates, 6 grams fat)

Maple Spiced Oatmeal with Currants

Bring 2 cups water to a boil. Add ½ cup steel-cut oats, reduce heat and cook for 20 minutes. Add ¼ cup currants during the last 10 minutes of cooking. When the oatmeal is done, add 1 tsp. gluten-free maple extract, 1tsp. cinnamon and ¼ tsp. of allspice

(215 calories, 7 grams protein, 41 grams carbohydrates, 3 grams fat)

Smoked Salmon and Egg Wraps

Preheat oven to 350 degrees. Scramble 3 egg whites with one egg and spoon egg mixture down the center of a whole-grain tortilla. Top with 1 ounce of smoked salmon and sprinkle with dill and 1/8 cup of Havarti cheese – fold up tortilla and bake in the oven seam side down for 5-10 minutes or until cheese melts.

(290 calories, 18 grams protein, 26 grams carbohydrates, 8 grams fat)

Pancakes with Strawberry Banana Sauce

These are quick to make!

In a blender, combine 2 cups fresh strawberries with 1 small banana and 1 tsp. honey. Pour into a bowl and set aside.

DO NOT WASH OUT THE BLENDER. Add ½ cup silken tofu, ½ cup soy milk or almond milk, 2 tbsp. ground flaxseed, ¾ cup almond flour, ½ cup

soy flour, 2 tsp. baking powder, sea salt and 1 egg.
Pour batter onto a hot griddle using 1 tbsp. of Grapeseed oil
(3 pancakes with ½ cup of sauce = 250 calories, 14 grams protein, 17 grams
carbohydrates, 2 grams fat)

Spinach Omelet with Canadian Bacon

Whisk together 3 egg whites with one egg, ¾ cup spinach, 1 slice Canadian
Bacon – chopped and pour into hot skillet on medium heat. Enjoy one slice
of bread, toasted (made from rice) with a tablespoon of almond butter on
top.
(540 calories, 25 grams protein, 55 grams carbohydrates, 12 grams fat)

Vegetable Frittata

Whisk together 1 cup egg whites with one egg, sea salt, pepper and
¼ cup shredded swiss cheese. In a hot skillet, cook 1 cup of your
favorite vegetables (peppers, onions, broccoli, mushrooms work
well) in 1 tablespoon of olive oil. Add egg white mixture and cook
until eggs are set. Serve with grilled tomatoes.
(250 calories, 12 grams protein, 22 grams carbohydrates, 7 grams fat)

Turkey Sausage and Asparagus Bake

Preheat oven to 400 degrees. Squeeze turkey out of sausage casing into a
medium hot skillet with 1 tablespoon of olive oil and cook through. Coat a
baking pan with cooking spray and sprinkle the sausage, ½ cup chopped
onion, 10 ounces of asparagus or broccoli. Beat 2 cups egg whites with 2
eggs, 2 cups soy milk or almond milk, ¼ cup Parmesan cheese, sea salt,
pepper and ½ tsp. dried tarragon. Pour over turkey mixture and bake for 20
minutes. Serve with sliced tomatoes.
(350 calories, 22 grams protein, 32 grams carbohydrates, 10 grams fat)

Blueberry Crunch Smoothie

In a blender, add 1 cup blueberries, ½ cup Kashi Go Lean Crunch, 1
container of 2x Protein Greek Yogurt (any flavor), 1 cup Almond milk or soy
milk, 1 tbsp. ground flaxseed and ice. Blend well
(375 calories, 25 grams protein, 32 grams carbohydrates, 8 grams fat)

Scrambled Egg Whites with Turkey Sausage and Tomatoes

Scramble 3 egg whites with one egg and sprinkle with 1/8 cup Parmesan cheese. Cook 2 turkey sausage links with sliced tomato.
(350 calories, 22 grams protein, 18 grams carbohydrates, 12 grams fat)

2 Poached Eggs, 2 Slices of Turkey Bacon, 1 tomato sliced and ½ cup strawberries dipped in ½ cup yogurt.

Poach eggs in egg poacher and cook turkey bacon and tomato slices in a skillet. Eat one yolk only.
(350 calories, 22 grams protein, 32 grams carbohydrates, 10 grams fat)

Eggs Florentine with Blueberries

Sauté 1 cup fresh spinach and pour 3 egg whites with one egg over spinach and scramble until set. Sprinkle with 2 tbsp. feta cheese. Enjoy with ½ cup blueberries.
(350 calories, 25 grams protein, 32 grams carbohydrates, 8 grams fat)

Chocolate Oatmeal

This may sound out of the ordinary for a weight loss breakfast but it is full of protein and will keep you going all morning. In a saucepan, combine 1/3 cup oats, ½ cup water and 1 scoop of Elite Chocolate Protein. Stir in 1 tbsp. of peanut butter.
(325 calories, 26 grams protein, 18 grams carbohydrates, 4 grams fat)

Denver Omelet

Cook ¼ red pepper- chopped, ¼ cup diced ham, 1 slice of onion, chopped in 1 tablespoon of olive oil. Add 3 egg whites with one egg to skillet and season with pepper. Fold over into an omelet. Serve with sliced tomatoes.
(325 calories, 28 grams protein, 32 grams carbohydrates, 8 grams fat)

Lunch Suggestions:

Edamame Salad with Chicken –

Grate 1 tsp. of orange zest in a bowl then add 2 tablespoons Rice Wine Vinegar, 1 tbsp. olive oil and 2 tbsp. chives. Whisk together and add 8 oz. of edamame, sliced cucumber, 1 cup cooked chicken and cut up the orange. Toss well.

(402 calories, 37 grams protein, 34 grams carbohydrates, 15 grams fat)

Barbecue Chicken Salad (without the grill)

In a bowl, whisk together ¼ cup barbecue sauce, 2 tbsp. cider vinegar, 1 tbsp. water and 2 tbsp. olive oil. Add 1 cup cooked chicken, 1 cup black beans, 1 tomato – chopped, 1/8 cup green chiles and Romaine lettuce

(400 calories, 29 grams protein, 42 grams carbohydrates, 13 grams fat)

Layered Gazpacho Salad

This is a quick and easy salad to prepare to take with you or whip up at home. For the Lemon-Garlic Vinaigrette, whisk together 1/8 cup red wine vinegar, ¼ olive oil, the juice of half a lemon, sea salt and pepper to taste, 1 tsp. minced garlic. Use a glass bowl if you have it and layer mixed lettuce greens, 2 tomatoes, ½ cucumber – sliced, ½ green or yellow pepper, ¼ cup chopped red onion and 2 hard-boiled eggs. Drizzle the dressing on top.

(350 calories, 18 grams protein, 28 grams carbohydrates, 12 grams fat)

Cashew Turkey Salad

Toss 2 cups mixed greens with 4 oz. of turkey breast (not deli meat), ½ cup of drained Mandarin oranges, 1 ½ tbsp. of low-fat honey mustard dressing, ½ tbsp. of orange marmalade and 2 tbsp. of cashew nuts.

(375 calories, 16 grams protein, 36 grams carbohydrates, 6 grams fat)

Tropical Tuna Salad

When you cook rice, make a batch and store in the fridge for a quick meal any time during the week. It will keep for up to 5 days in an air-tight container.

Mix 1 cup brown rice, ½ cup vanilla yogurt and 1 tablespoon of pineapple juice (from draining 1 can pineapple tidbits in juice) Fold in ½ cup mango, ½ cup pineapple and 1 can tuna (drained) into rice mixture. Sprinkle with

toasted coconut. (Cook 1 tbsp. shredded coconut in a skillet for 6 minutes until golden brown stirring frequently)
(250 calories, 15 grams protein, 41 grams carbohydrates, 3 grams fat)

Chicken Couscous Salad with Yogurt Curry Dressing

Make a batch of couscous or brown rice and store in fridge for quick meals any day of the week. Combine 1 cup couscous, 1 cup cooked chicken, 1 cup garbanzo beans, 1 green onion – chopped, ½ red pepper – chopped. Toss with Yogurt Curry Dressing: Mix ½ cup plain yogurt, 1 tablespoon olive oil, sea salt and ¼ tsp. curry powder and toss with couscous mixture. Serve over a bed of lettuce.
(325 calories, 22 grams protein, 32 grams carbohydrates, 7 grams fat)

Beef, Lettuce and Tomato Wraps

Toss 1 cup lean roast beef with a pinch of chili powder, sea salt, 1 tsp. oregano and 1 tsp. cumin and place in a whole-grain tortilla. Add lettuce and tomatoes and ¼ cup plain yogurt mixed with a pinch of horseradish.
(325 calories, 29 grams protein, 24 grams carbohydrates, 8 grams fat)

Egg Hummus Salad

Take 4 hard-boiled eggs and cut out 2 of the yolks – chop the rest. Add ½ cup celery, 2 tbsp. of chipotle-flavored hummus, 2 tbsp. low-fat mayonnaise and mix well. Serve over a bed of leafy greens with grape-size tomatoes
(330 calories, 17 grams protein, 35 grams carbohydrates, 10 grams fat)

Chicken Fajita Salad

Many grocery stores offer pre-cooked fajita chicken strips. Add to a bed of mixed greens with your favorite vegetables like red pepper, onion, tomatoes, etc. Mix together 1/3 cup Italian dressing with ¼ cup plain yogurt. Drizzle over salad.
(300 calories, 26 grams protein, 18 grams carbohydrates, 10 grams fat)

Curry Chicken Salad in Tomatoes

This makes a beautiful presentation if you are having friends over for lunch.

Combine 2 cups cooked chicken in pieces, 1 cup diced celery, 1 apple – diced, ½ cup raisins, ¼ cup low-fat mayonnaise, 2 tablespoons mango chutney, 1 tbsp. plain yogurt, juice of half a lime, 1 tsp. curry powder and ½ tsp. ground cumin. Slice the top off of a large tomato and scoop out the inside. Scoop the chicken salad into the tomato halves and serve on a bed of lettuce.

(1 cup chicken salad in a tomato = 350 calories, 22 grams protein, 34 grams carbohydrates, 6 grams fat)

Turkey Sandwich with lettuce and tomatoes on bread made from rice

Spread mustard on one piece of rice bread and 1 tablespoon of Miracle Whip on the other piece. Add sliced turkey breast, lettuce and tomato.

(325 calories, 26 grams protein, 32 grams carbohydrates, 6 grams fat)

Crab Seafood Pasta Salad

Use bowtie pasta made from rice and prepare as directed. Combine 1 cup crabmeat, 1 carrot – sliced, ½ cup celery- chopped, 1 diced tomato, ¼ cup low-fat Italian dressing, pepper and the juice of one lemon. Add the drained pasta to the crab mixture and mix well. Serve over a bed of lettuce.

(350 calories, 28 grams protein, 36 grams carbohydrates, 6 grams fat)

Chicken Quesadillas with Pesto

Spread one whole-grain tortilla with 2 tablespoons of pesto. Place cooked grilled chicken strips on one half of the tortilla. Add sliced Italian tomato, 2 tablespoons of julienned sun-dried tomatoes and sprinkle ½ cup low-fat Italian mixed shredded cheese. Fold over tortilla and coat a hot skillet with cooking spray. Cook about 2-3 minutes on each side. Remove and serve with one tablespoon of low-fat yogurt or low-fat sour cream for dipping.

(350 calories, 26 grams protein, 32 grams carbohydrates, 7 grams fat)

Tuna Apple Salad

Combine 1 can tuna- drained, ½ cup diced onion, ½ cup diced celery, 1 tbsp. dill relish, 1 tsp. Dijon Mustard, 2 tbsp. plain yogurt or low-fat mayo, and 1 apple – diced. Serve over a bed of lettuce with sliced tomatoes.

(375 calories, 26 grams protein, 32 grams carbohydrates, 6 grams fat)

Dinner suggestions:

Chicken Quinoa Spaghetti with Broccoli Pesto

Use whole-grain pasta or pasta made from rice or quinoa and cook according to package directions. Drain. Steam 1 bag of frozen chopped broccoli in a steamer – not the bag. In a food processor, puree broccoli, 1 cup vegetable broth, ¼ cup Parmesan, 2 tbsp. olive oil, 1 clove garlic and sea salt. Toss pasta, 4 cups cooked chicken and broccoli pesto together and season with pepper to taste.

(498 calories, 37 grams protein, 57 grams carbohydrates, 15 grams fat)

Sesame Shrimp with Asparagus and Basmati Rice

Cook rice according to label directions. Toss Asparagus in 1 tbsp. olive oil, 1 tsp. sesame oil and sprinkle sea salt and garlic powder. Place on a large cookie sheet and Bake in the oven at 400 degrees for 10 minutes. In a small bowl, whisk together 3 tablespoons reduced-sodium soy sauce, 2 tsp. rice wine vinegar, 1 green onion, chopped and ½ sesame oil. Set aside. Heat a large skillet with 1 tbsp. olive oil and add 1 pound shrimp, 1/8 tsp. crushed red pepper. Cook until shrimp are opaque. Serve shrimp with rice and asparagus.

(535 calories, 34 grams protein, 57 grams carbohydrates, 12 grams fat)

Simple Grilled Chicken Breasts with Pistachio Basil Pesto, Pan-Roasted Red Potatoes and Tossed Salad with Mustard Vinaigrette

Napoli di Classico makes an excellent, all-natural pesto available in the tomato sauce section of most grocery stores if you do not want to make pesto from scratch.

(615 calories, 34 grams protein, 42 grams carbs, 15 grams fat)

~ Here are the recipes for this simple and delicious menu ~

Pistachio Basil Pesto

Preheat your oven to 350 degrees. Place 8 oz. of pistachio nuts and 4 oz. of pine nuts on a cookie sheet and bake for 6-7 minutes. Remove to a plate and cool. In a food processor, combine nuts, 1 cup fresh basil, 2 garlic cloves, ¾ cup olive oil, sea salt and pepper to taste.

Pan-Roasted Red Potatoes

If the potatoes are real small, you can leave them whole, otherwise, cut them in half. Toss with 1 ½ pounds (or about a fistful for each person) with ¼ cup olive oil, 1 tsp. garlic powder, 1 tablespoon Italian Herb Seasoning, sea salt and pepper to taste. Roast in the oven at 350 for about 45 minutes.

Simple Grilled Chicken Filets

You can purchase thin chicken filets in the grocery store and they are always convenient to have on hand. Sprinkle each breast with sea salt and lemon pepper. Heat 1 tablespoon of olive oil in a skillet and cook each chicken breast about 3-5 minutes on each side.
Serve with Pesto on the side or spread some on each chicken breast.

Mustard Vinaigrette

2 tbsp. of fresh lemon juice
2 tsp. Dijon mustard
1 tsp. minced garlic
Sea salt and pepper to taste
6 tablespoons extra-virgin olive oil

Whisk together all the ingredients and place in an air-tight container. Toss with your favorite leafy greens, tomatoes, cucumbers, etc. for a delicious salad for dinner.

Turkey Black Bean Chili with Tossed Salad in a Peanut Butter Vinaigrette

Cook 1 pound ground turkey in a large skillet – drain if necessary. Add 2 cups black beans, 1 1/2 cup salsa, 2 Italian tomato – chopped, 2 tsp. chili powder and 1 tsp. ground cumin and bring to a low boil. Simmer for 15-20 minutes.

Peanut Butter Vinaigrette

Whisk together 1 tablespoon peanut butter, 1/8 cup rice wine vinegar, 1 tbsp. sesame oil, ¼ cup olive oil, 1 tsp. honey, 1 tsp. cayenne pepper, 1 tsp. ground ginger, sea salt and pepper to taste. Toss with your favorite mixed greens and add toasted walnuts, ¼ cup Parmesan, tomatoes, cucumbers, ¼ chopped red onion

(630 calories, 28 grams protein, 42 grams carbohydrates, 8 grams fat)

Rotisserie Chicken with Roasted Vegetables and Lemon Pepper Couscous

Pick up a Rotisserie Chicken at the grocery store and serve with roasted vegetables from earlier and make couscous according to label directions and season with lemon pepper.

(470 calories, 28 grams protein, 42 grams carbohydrates, 6 grams fat)

Honey-Mustard Pork Tenderloin with Sweet Potato Fries and Steamed Broccoli with lemon

Preheat oven to 375 degrees. Mix together 1 tbsp. honey, 1 tbsp. mustard, 1 tsp. sea salt, ¼ tsp. ground allspice and a pinch of cayenne pepper. Coat a pork tenderloin and roast in the oven for 45 minutes. Remove and let stand for 10 minutes covered. Place pan on burner and add ¼ cup water and 1 tablespoon of brown sugar. Mix well scraping bottom of pan. Drizzle sauce over pork.

Sweet Potato Fries – Toss sliced sweet potatoes in olive oil, sea salt and pepper and roast in oven with pork tenderloin. Steam broccoli and serve with lemon

(675 calories, 28 grams protein, 32 grams carbohydrates, 6 grams fat)

Grilled Halibut with Lime and Cilantro Bulgur Pilaf and Garlic Green Beans

Mix together the juice of one lime, 1 tbsp. cilantro, 1 tsp. olive oil and 1 clove garlic – chopped. Coat halibut in mixture and let stand while you make the Bulgur Pilaf. Cook ½ cup slivered almonds in 2 tbsp. canola oil about 2 minutes – remove. Add 1 more tablespoon of canola oil, ½ cup chopped onion and ½ cup shredded carrots and cook until crisp-tender. Stir in 1 can low-sodium chicken or vegetable broth, 1 cup bulgur, 1 tsp. lemon pepper and sea salt. Cover and simmer for 15 minutes. Steam green beans and sprinkle with garlic powder while you cook halibut in a hot skillet about 10-20 minutes turning once.

(445 calories, 28 grams protein, 32 grams carbohydrates, 12 grams fat)

Sweet and Sour Shrimp with Brown Rice and Asparagus

Cook brown rice according to label directions and season with sea salt and pepper. In large skillet, cook asparagus with 1 tbsp. olive oil, sea salt and pepper. Heat a skillet on medium heat and add 1 tablespoon olive oil and 1 red pepper – chopped and cook for 3-5 minutes. Add 1/3 cup apricot jam, 2 tsp. red wine vinegar and 1 cup cooked shrimp. Heat through about 2 minutes and serve over rice with asparagus.

(495 calories, 21 grams protein, 45 grams carbohydrates, 6 grams fat)

Chicken Teriyaki Skillet Dinner

In a large skillet, add 1 ½ tbsp. olive oil on medium heat and 2 cups chicken pieces. Season with sea salt and pepper and stir-fry until no longer pink in the center - remove from skillet. Add another tablespoon of oil to skillet and add 2 carrots – chopped and 1 zucchini chopped. Add 2 tbsp. low-sodium Teriyaki sauce and stir well. Sprinkle with ½ cup chopped green onions and ½ cup Parmesan. Serve with brown rice.

(534 calories, 31 grams protein, 28 grams carbohydrates, 8 grams fat)

Sesame Beef Stir Fry with Brown Rice

This recipe is a great way to use broccoli slaw available in the produce section of most grocery stores. Cook brown rice according to label directions. While the rice is cooking, brown 1 pound of lean ground beef in a large skillet. Drain and set aside. In the same skillet, add 1 tbsp. sesame oil, broccoli slaw, 1 cup napa cabbage, 2 cloves garlic, minced and 3 green onions – diced. Add one cup of the brown rice and 2 tbsp. low-sodium soy sauce. Return the cooked ground beef to the skillet and season with red pepper flakes to taste.
(410 calories, 28 grams protein, 42 g. carbs, 10 grams fat)

Balsamic-Glazed Chicken with Pine Nut Couscous and Broccoli
Mix 3 tbsp. balsamic vinegar, 2 tbsp. olive oil, 2 tbsp. fresh rosemary – chopped, pepper and 3 cloves garlic – minced. Coat chicken in mixture. Cook couscous according to label directions. In a large skillet, add one tablespoon of olive oil and cook chicken breasts about 6-7 minutes on each side. Steam broccoli and keep warm. Toast pine nuts in a small skillet for about 1-2 minutes and sprinkle over all to serve.
(500 calories, 28 grams protein, 32 grams carbohydrates, 8 grams fat)

Chicken Fajitas
Cook 1 red pepper, 1 green pepper and one onion in a skillet with 2 tablespoons of olive oil until caramelized. Add 2 cups fajita-seasoned chicken strips to skillet and heat through. Warm 2 whole-grain tortillas or 2 corn tortillas in the oven or in the microwave and serve with plain, low-fat yogurt and low-fat shredded cheddar cheese
(535 calories, 28 grams protein, 35 grams carbohydrates, 10 grams fat)

Tuscan Style Grilled Chicken with Angel Hair Pasta and Salad
Sprinkle chicken breasts with sea salt and pepper and cook in 1 ½ tablespoons of olive oil until no longer pink. Cut up 2 Italian tomatoes and toss with fresh basil, 1 garlic clove, minced and 1 tablespoon of olive oil. Cook fresh angel hair pasta and drain. Toss with tomato mixture. Serve with a side salad for a complete meal.
(565 calories, 28 grams protein, 35 grams carbohydrates, 8 grams fat)

Dinner: Buffalo Burgers with Cole Slaw and Baked Fries
Season buffalo meat with low-sodium Lawry's Seasoned Salt or another
favorite beef seasoning - form into patties and cook on the grill outside or in
a hot skillet. Wash 4 potatoes and slice into steak fries. Place in bowl and
toss with 2 tablespoons Italian seasoning, sea salt and pepper. Place potato
wedges on cookie sheet and bake in the oven at 400 degrees for 45 minutes.
Toss packaged coleslaw mix with ½ cup low-fat mayonnaise, 2 tbsp.
vinegar, 1 tablespoon honey and ¼ of an onion, chopped.
(529 calories, 28 grams protein, 36 grams carbohydrates, 3 grams fat)

Snack suggestions:
It is important to have emergency foods on hand at home, in your car, purse,
brief case and at the office when hunger pangs strike. It will allow you to
make smart food choices instead of pulling into your local drive-thru or eat
junk food that lacks nutrients.

Anytime Snack Mix
Preheat the oven to 400 degrees. Mix together, ¼ cup each of almonds,
cashews, pecans, walnuts and sunflower seeds. Bake for 5 minutes. Cool
and add 6 tablespoons dried organic cranberries and golden raisins and mix
well.
(1/4 cup serving = 213 calories, 5 grams protein, 20 grams carbohydrates, 10
grams fat)

Strawberry Tofu Smoothie
In a blender, add 1 cup organic strawberries, 1 cup 2x protein Greek Yogurt,

¼ cup water, 1 tsp. vanilla extract and ice. Blend well
(175 calories, 12 grams protein, 15 grams carbohydrates, 3 grams fat)

Baked Fruit

This recipe is quick and easy if you are at home. Cut up fresh fruit like apples, pears, peaches, plums or apricots to equal 4 cups. Drizzle with a tablespoon of balsamic vinegar and ¼ tsp. cardamom. Bake at 375 degrees for 15 minutes. Sprinkle with toasted almonds or pecans for some added protein.
(215 calories, 6 grams protein with nuts, 30 grams carbohydrates, 3 grams fat)

Salmon-Spinach Pinwheels

Use up the rest of the salmon and dill from the morning for this quick snack. Mix 1 pkg. of reduced-fat cream cheese with 1 tbsp. of dill and spread over a whole-grain tortilla. Add 2 ounces of salmon, 4 spinach leaves and 4 red bell pepper strips.
(2 pinwheels = 130 calories, 6 grams protein, 14 grams carbohydrates, 6 grams fat)

Guacamole with Baked Rice Chips

Mash 2 ripe avocadoes with ½ cup diced red onion, 1 Italian tomato, ½ cup chopped cilantro, 1 tsp. minced jalapeno, 1 tsp. lime juice and sea salt to taste. Mix well and serve with chips made from rice available at health food stores.
(1/2 cup serving with chips = 215 calories, 2 grams protein, 12 grams carbohydrates, 6 grams fat)

Black bean Dip with baked rice tortilla chips

(1/2 cup dip with 8 chips = 195 calories, 8 grams protein, 20 grams carbohydrates, 6 grams fat)

Handful of almonds or mixed nuts with an apple
(225 calories, 4 grams protein, 12 grams carbohydrates, 8 grams fat)

Roasted Vegetable Dip with Baked Rice Chips
Roasting vegetables is a great way to add flavor without a lot of fat. The dip stores well in the fridge and the vegetables make a great addition to dinner. Preheat oven to 400 degrees. Cut up 1 zucchini, 1 yellow squash, 1 red pepper, 1 small onion and 1 clove of garlic. Toss them with 2 tablespoons extra-virgin olive oil, sea salt and pepper. Bake in the oven for 30 minutes. Remove and place vegetables into a food processor and blend for 1 minute. Serve warm with baked rice chips. (You can triple the recipe so you have roasted vegetables for dinner)
(1/2 cup dip with 8 rice chips =115 calories, 3 grams protein, 15 grams carbohydrates, 2 grams fat)

Fruit Parfait
Alternate fresh fruit like strawberries, blueberries and raspberries in a parfait glass with 1 cup Strawberry Greek Yogurt
(175 calories, 8 grams protein, 26 grams carbohydrates, 5 grams fat)

½ cup of Roasted soy nuts with 2 tablespoons of raisins
(175 calories, 8 grams protein, 18 grams carbohydrates, 7 grams fat)

Kiwi-Banana Smoothie
In a blender, add 1 kiwi (peeled), ½ banana, 1 tablespoon peanut butter and 1 carton of 2x protein Greek Yogurt (any flavor). Blend well
(195 calories, 8 grams protein, 15 grams carbohydrates, 3 grams fat)

Roasted Nut Snack with Apple
Preheat oven to 350 degrees. Toss 1 cup mixed nuts with 1 ½ tbsp. apple cider and ½ tsp. celery salt or you can use curry powder. Spread on a cookie sheet and bake for 4-6 minutes. Enjoy warm with an apple.
(a handful of nuts with apple = 285 calories, 5 grams protein, 15 grams

carbohydrates, 10 grams fat)

1 Pink Lady Apple dipped in almond butter

(225 calories, 8 grams protein, 15 grams carbohydrates, 4 grams fat)

½ cup cottage cheese with ½ cup edamame or handful of nuts

(215 calories, 18 grams protein, 5 grams carbohydrates, 8 grams fat)

Toasted Pumpkin Seeds with Romaine and Avocado

This is something you can whip up for a satisfying snack when at home. Toast ½ cup pumpkin seeds in a skillet for about 3 minutes. Remove and let cool. In a bowl, add 1 cup Romaine lettuce, ¼ of an avocado - sliced, 1 chopped tomato, 1 green onion – chopped and ½ of a red pepper, sliced. Toss in a **Lime Vinaigrette** made with juice of a lime, ¼ cup cilantro, 1 tsp. minced garlic, sea salt and pepper to taste, 6 tbsp. of olive oil.

(315 calories, 6 grams protein, 11 grams carbohydrates, 4 grams fat)

Cream of Rice with Toasted Almonds

Combine 4 tablespoons of Cream of Rice, 1 scoop of Elite Whey Protein and ¾ cup water in a saucepan. Stir and cook for about 3 minutes or until thickened. Sprinkle with cinnamon and slivered almonds.

(225 calories, 22 grams protein, 18 grams carbohydrates, 3 grams fat)

2 hard-boiled eggs and an orange – discard one yolk

(195 calories, 22 grams protein, 15 grams carbohydrates, 6 grams fat)

Grocery Shopping List

PROTEIN SOURCES

4-5 Servings per day
Eggs - 1 whole egg with 3-4 egg whites
Egg Whites only – 4-6

FISH – Salmon, Tuna, Halibut, Cod, Orange Roughy, Tilapia

Shellfish – 3 oz. limit 1-2 servings per week
Chicken Breast or Turkey Breast – about the size of a deck of cards

Lean Beef – Buffalo, Venison, Lamb
Tofu – 1 cup limited to 4 times per week
Tempeh 3 oz.

GLYCEMIC INDEX AND WHY IT MATTERS

LOW GLYCEMIC VEGETABLES – Servings per day = unlimited
Eat fresh or frozen vegetables, organic when possible – stay away from canned vegetables

Aspragus
Artichokes
Bean Sprouts
Bell Peppers
Broccoli
Brussel Sprouts
Cauliflower
Celery
Cucumber
Cabbage – red, green, Chinese
Onions – chives, leeks, garlic
Green Beans
Mushrooms
Okra
Radishes
Snow peas
Sprouts
Salsa – sugar-free
Tomatoes
Water chestnuts – 5 whole
Squash – zucchini, yellow or spaghetti
Kelps – all types – dulce, walkami, nori
Greens – bok choy, escarole, spinach, dandelion, mustard, beet
Mixed Greens - Romaine, Red and Green Leaf, Endive, Arugula, Radicchio,

Watercress, Chicory

HIGH GLYCEMIC VEGETABLES
Servings per day = 1
Serving Size = ½ cup - best eaten with a protein source

Beets
Carrots = 12 baby carrots, 2 raw or ½ cup cooked
Winter squash = acorn or butternut
Potatoes – sweet potatoes, yams, russet, white or red

OILS
4 Servings per day
Serving Size = 1 tsp.
Oils should not be cold pressed

Flaxseed oil – refrigerate
Walnut oil
Extra Virgin Olive oil
Canola Oil
Sesame Oil
Olives – ripe or green - limit 8
Avocado - ¼ of a whole one
Mayonnaise made with canola oil
Butter – 1 tsp.

WHOLE GRAINS – no wheat or gluten
Servings per day = 2
Serving Size = ½ cup

Amaranth
Teff
Quinoa
Rice – basmati, brown, wild
Corn Tortillas- no more than 2

PASTA – preferably made from rice or corn instead of wheat
Limit to 2-3 servings per week

Breads = 1 slice made from rice or gluten-free
Crackers = 3 crackers gluten-free
Cereals = ½ cup free from gluten, wheat and dairy

LEGUMES

Servings per day =1-2
Servings Size = ½ cup cooked
Beans – Garbanzo, Pinto, Fat-free refried, Black, Lima, Cannellini, Navy, Mung, Hummus (1/4 cup)
Green Soy Beans – Edamame
Peas – yellow and green split peas, sweet green peas
Lentils – red and green
Bean Soups

FRUIT

Servings per day = 1-2

Apple – 1 medium
Apricot – 1 medium
Blackberries ½ cup
Blueberries ½ cup
Raspberries - 1 cup
Strawberries – 1 cup
Cherries – ½ cup
Grapes – ½ cup
Melon – ½ Cantaloupe, ¼ Honeydew
Nectarine – 2 small
Peach – 2 small
Kiwi – 2 small
Tangerine – 2 small
Plum – 3 small
Mango
Papaya

NUTS and SEEDS

Servings per day = 2

Almonds – whole – 10-15
Hazelnuts – 10-15

Natural Nut Butters – 1 tablespoon
Peanuts – 9-12
Sunflower – 2 tablespoons
Pumpkin – 2 tablespoons
Sesame Seeds –2 tablespoons

BEVERAGES
Unlimited
Coffee –
Teas
Purified Water
Mineral Water – plain or flavored unsweetened

Preparing Your Kitchen

There is definitely a relationship between nutrition and the mind including emotions that help determine an optimum diet. In order to insure mental and emotional well-being:

> The diet must consist of **un-processed, whole foods.**

> **Foods that rob the body** of nutrients need to be **eliminated** to maintain nutritional balance crucial to mental and emotional stability.

> Foods that leave heavy, toxic by-products in the bloodstream must not be eaten to **avoid poisoning** the body and the mind.

> Foods should be eaten in a **calm, harmonious environment** in a relaxed disposition.

> You should eat when you are hungry for fuel, **not for stimulation** or a means of "escape."

*Perhaps the most pressing need is the **elimination of all 'nonfood' items** from the diet. These nonfoods include white sugar, white flour, alcohol, salt, condiments, and all heavily processed foods. These foods alone are the major causes of mental and emotional illnesses, and they perform no positive function in the body whatsoever.*

Fat Loss Supplements

Two-thirds of Americans are overweight and one-third is considered obese. The interest in weight loss is apparent when you walk into your local health food store and find a category labeling endless shelves of supplements promising to help you lose weight. There is no substitute for increased activity with complete, mini-meals every 3-4 hours for achieving and maintaining your ideal weight however there are some nutritional supplements that may help:

GREEN TEA – studies have shown that those drinking green tea or taking a green tea supplement combined with healthy meals and exercise lose more weight compared to those who do not take anything at all. The other health benefits to green tea is it helps to lower cholesterol, triglycerides, appetite-suppressing hormone leptin and cortisol, the stress hormone.

CHROMIUM PICOLINATE – (500 mcg.) is an excellent supplement to stabilize blood sugar levels throughout the day that help you avoid increased hunger. If you are diabetic, diagnosed with diabetes and/or taking insulin, please check with your doctor first before taking this supplement as it makes insulin work much more efficiently. Another added benefit to this supplement is it helps lower cholesterol naturally.

5-HTP – (5-hydroxytryptophan) boosts levels of serotonin, a neurotransmitter involved in mood and appetite. The dose used in research of 5-HTP is 50-100 mg once or twice a day, taken between meals. Do NOT take this supplement if you are on any anti-depressant.

CLA (Conjugated Linoleic Acid) – is wonderful for helping to get rid of abdominal fat. One of the best CLA supplements is Tonalin with a recommended dose of 3,000 – 4,000 mg. daily.

RESVERATROL – is phytonutrient found in red wine that is getting quite a bit of attention in the media as an anti-aging supplement. Scientists in Germany found it inhibits fat storage and the development of new fat cells. The recommended dosage is 100-150 mg. daily.

GROUND FLAXSEED or FIBER – helps keep you full and slows the release of glucose in the bloodstream preventing blood sugar highs and lows that trigger cravings for junk food. Another benefit for women is ground flaxseed has lignans which attach themselves to excess estrogen receptor sites in the body helping to eliminate them. Estrogen dominance can occur as a woman approaches and goes through menopause. One-eighth of a cup is all you need – add it to oatmeal, sprinkle it on salads or add it to a smoothie in a blender.

DHEA – is a natural counter-regulator of cortisol and assists in abdominal weight loss plus it helps improve insulin sensitivity. The usual starting dosage is 50 mg. for men and 25 mg. for women however, DHEA is NOT recommended for anyone with prostate, breast or ovarian cancer. Blood levels should be tested every 3 months.

CALCIUM – numerous studies link calcium intake with a reduced risk of obesity so make sure you are getting at least 1,000 mg daily of this very important mineral. The best way to take calcium is to take 500 mg. of calcium with 250 mg. of magnesium in the morning and again at night about an hour before bedtime. It helps lower blood pressure naturally and will help you get a good night's sleep.

Fat Loss for the Fast and Furious
(For Queens on the go all the time)

Have you tried every diet on the planet? Do you exercise, drink water, do all the things you should be doing to lose weight and still can't lose a pound? Are you frustrated beyond belief? Here are some simple rules that will help you look great without going on a strict diet or feeling deprived.

1. **Eat from the earth** - make a point of eating more whole foods from the produce section instead of foods that come in a box or bag. Not only will you taste the difference, you will notice the difference in your waistline as you will stay full longer. If you are in a hurry, check out HYPERLINK "http://www.regenerationusa.com" www.regenerationusa.com for an excellent whole food bar as seen on Good Morning America.

2. **Eliminate soft drinks** – Unfortunately, there is nothing good to say about soft drinks, regular or diet, it doesn't matter. They both do a disservice to your health and body. Invest in a water filter for your home, ice and lots of lemons. Eventually, filtered lemon water will be all you want to drink.

3. **Eat soup before your meals** - soup will give you a full feeling due to the combination of liquids and solids and you will lower your calorie intake by about 20% every single day.

4. **Practice good posture sitting or standing** - lift your head up high, pull those abs in, chin up and you will automatically look slimmer. Plus this added effort does burn calories.

5. **Beware of salads with all the trimmings** - of course you should order a salad whenever possible, however, be aware by the time they have added the cheese, egg, bacon, croutons and salad dressing, the calories are quite high. Order the dressing on the side and eliminate the bacon, cheese and croutons and you will reduce your caloric intake dramatically.

6. **Take time out to exercise** - schedule it, do whatever you can to make exercise a part of your daily routine. You will feel less stressed and you will lose weight.

7. **Eat some probiotics** - this means Greek yogurt which has 3 times more probiotics in it than regular yogurt to improve digestion.

8. **Laugh -** it really is the best medicine. It will strengthen your immune system, reduce food cravings, help increase your threshold for pain and reduce the amount of cortisol (stress hormone) released throughout your body.

Following these simple rules will help you look and feel better, and happy in your own skin without going on a strict diet. You still need to find time for exercise and find foods that you like and can live with. Make some simple changes like switching to mayonnaise made with olive oil. Use olive oil instead of butter and switch to soy or almond milk instead of regular milk. These changes can make all the difference when it comes to

Fat Loss Contingency Planning

Gaining weight can be so frustrating. Certainly huge portions, decadent meals and desserts, wine and sugary soft drinks will lead to weight gain If you are eating healthy foods and exercising on a regular basis and still packing on the pounds, something else must be going on inside the body.

Here are 5 factors to consider that can cause weight gain:

Lack of Sleep – when you are tired, it is difficult to handle stressful situations throughout the day and you may be reaching for food to cope with the fatigue, lack of energy or if you feel a bit irritable.

Lack of nutrient-dense meals every 3-4 hours– when the body is lacking nutrients or goes way too long without food, it will cause huge fluctuations in blood sugar levels and that can lead to bingeing on larger than normal meals, cravings and inflammation throughout the body.

Prescription medications for blood pressure, cholesterol, depression, headaches or whatever can actually cause the body to gain weight from a modest amount up to ten pounds per month. Sometimes simply feeling better on anti-depressants can cause the appetite to increase.

Thyroid function – hypothyroidism is becoming rampant in this country that is a deficiency in the thyroid hormone. This can cause a decrease in metabolism causing weight gain.

Peri-Menopause to Post-Menopause – this change can happen to women at any age which causes a loss of estrogen leading to weight gain. Lifting weights is one of the best ways to counteract the effects of estrogen imbalance.

Food Sensitivities

There is an interesting story about a family who followed a healthy diet of mostly fruits, vegetables, nuts and seeds for several years. The children were well behaved, kind and gracious to their parents as well as each other with no signs of being irritable or cranky.

One day, their mother fed her children several slices of whole-wheat bread and within an hour, the children were fighting amongst themselves and had several outbursts of anger and emotional tantrums. You might think this is a coincidence, however the point is a pure, high quality diet has a profound effect on mental and emotional states.

Studies have shown that eating foods high in fat tends to dull the mind and cloud thinking. Digesting fat is so demanding on the body that blood is diverted away from the brain to the digestive system and as a result, thinking processes become slower and depression can occur.

Although Western science has only recently discovered the relationship between mental states and nutrition, people in the Eastern countries have been aware of the effects of diet on the mind since around 4000 B.C. Foods can be classified into three types:

Pure Foods – which consist of primarily fresh fruits and vegetables and have been shown to bring calmness and tranquility to the mind - pure foods are very important for those desiring spiritual growth and a meditative mind.

Stimulating Foods – include spices, meat, eggs, onions etc. cause a restless, unsatisfied state of mind and contribute to nervous disorders and emotional outbreaks.

Impure Foods – are highly processed with lots of preservatives that decrease thinking capacity, dull the senses and contribute to chronic mental ailments like accelerate the aging process and can cause an early death.

Basically, foods affect our mental and emotional state in two ways:

They either furnish or deplete vital nutrients upon which our mental and emotional health depend, and

They either do or do not produce toxic by-products in the body that poison the brain and contribute to emotional problems.

For example, eating grapes furnishes the blood with readily-assimilated natural sugars and minerals that are conducive to mental activity; consuming white sugar, on the other hand, depletes the body of B-vitamins, and this leads to nervousness and mental depression. Eating fresh raw foods places little or no toxic matter in the body; whereas eating preserved and cooked foods saturates the bloodstream with toxins that poison the body and interfere with brain function. Symptoms include:

Headaches

Insomnia

Fatigue

Irritability

Restlessness

Crying spells

Nervous breakdowns

Excessive worry

Inability to concentrate

Depression

Forgetfulness

Suicidal thoughts

Illogical fears

Allergies

Caffeine found in coffee, tea, cola drinks and chocolate, causes nervous disturbances, including anxiety. One to three cups of coffee contain enough caffeine to cause anxiety and other emotional disturbances. Caffeine also stimulates insulin secretion, thereby disturbing the blood-sugar level in the body.

Alcohol, too, disturbs the blood-sugar level. In fact, low blood sugar occurs in 70-90% of all alcoholics. As a result of studies, it was also discovered that most alcoholics suffer from a niacin (vitamin B3) deficiency that leads to periods of depression and feelings of lack of self-worth. Such emotional states may then lead to more alcohol drinking in an effort to escape these feelings.

All of the above-mentioned nutritional robbers tend to be self-perpetuating; that is, they create the very conditions that often make the user of these items return to them. For example – a withdrawal symptom caused by a lack of caffeine from not drinking coffee can be stopped by drinking another cup of coffee. The irritability caused by smoking is soothed by another cigarette. The "shakes" caused by a period of sobriety can be removed by another slug of whiskey.

The crashing blood-sugar levels created by sugar intake can be temporarily raised again by consuming another candy bar or other sugary "food." In short, all of these nonfood items are actually *addictive drugs* just as opium and heroin are. If we are truly concerned about the "drug problem" in America, it would be best if we set our own house in order first. This would remove the cause of many of our mental and emotional problems that result from faulty nutrition.

Day-To-Day Tips for Work and Home

Why We Eat What We Eat – The first step in changing the way you think about 'eating well' is to become aware of it.
SAD (Standard American Diet) shaped by fat, sugar and salt
The Business of Food – food manufacturer's produce food so you keep coming back – shelf life
Technology has changed what we eat - Potatoes used to be baked, boiled, or mashed; the labor involved in peeling, cutting, and cooking French fries meant that few home cooks served them, the economists point out. But now factories prepare potatoes for frying and ship them to fast-food outlets or freeze them for microwave cooking at home.

Can Healthy Eating be Satisfying? The answer is a resounding "YES!" – teach yourself to prepare food in a new paradigm. It can be so exciting!
Food can be satisfying
Vegetables are stimulating
Taste, Texture and Aroma

Shifting your Paradigm – You will be surprised to see the wide variety of delicious and satisfying foods that you can eat.
Retrain Your Brain
Moderation is Key
New skills

Other Tips:

Chew gum if you can do it without appearing unprofessional. Fat Loss Queen recommendation is a sugar free gum. Satisfies your urge to chew and the strong flavor especially mint keeps your taste buds occupied. Sugar free gum sweetened with xylitol would be the best. It keeps the cavity causing bacteria away.

Take stock of your environment

Any food items that might tempt your willpower should be kept out of sight, and even better out of the house or environment if possible. The adage " out of sight, out of mind " is true.

At work keep any candies in opaque containers so no visual temptation.

Even if you have been on every 'diet' in the world or gone on the roller-coaster ride of yo-yo dieting, you can succeed once and for all. Whether you want to lose weight, improve your health, looks or increase energy, this book will help you achieve your goals.

You will be able to transform your body and discover what really works for you. Too many of the 'diet' plans available are too restrictive, not realistic and leave you feeling starved and discouraged. My goal for you is to get your strength and fitness levels back, see results and change the way you think about weight loss.

No weight loss plan works without good nutrition and this book shows you the foods to eat, when to eat and how to turn yourself into a fat-burning machine instead of a fat-storing machine. When you create meals around the whole foods suggested in this book, you will create a whole new body in the process.

www.ingramcontent.com/pod-product-compliance
Lightning Source LLC
Chambersburg PA
CBHW080741290526

45790CB00008B/3280